Fat Girl

fat giRL

one woman's way out

Lived, Composed, and
Illustrated by
Irene O'Garden

HarperSan Francisco
A Division of HarperCollins *Publishing*

HarperSanFrancisco and the author, in association with the Rainforest Action Network, will facilitate the planting of two trees for every one tree used in the manufacture of this book.

HarperCollins books may be purchased for educational, business, or sales promotional use. For information, please call or write: Special Markets Department, HarperCollins Publishers, 10 East 53rd Street, New York, NY 10022.
Telephone: (212) 207-7528. Fax: (212) 207-7222.

FIRST HARPERCOLLINS CLOTH EDITION PUBLISHED IN 1993

ISBN 0–06–250727–3 (pbk. : alk paper)
Library of Congress Catalog Number 92–54663

93   94   95   96   97   ❖ HAD   10   9   8   7   6   5   4   3   2   1
This edition is printed on acid-free paper that meets the American National Standards Institute Z39.48 Standard.

I dedicate this book to anyone who is afraid to read it.

Awareness is Omnipotent.
Nothing in the universe can stop Her.
Awareness is Omnipotent.
Everything leads to Her.
Nothing is beneath Her.
Nothing is beyond Her.
Nothing but Herself.

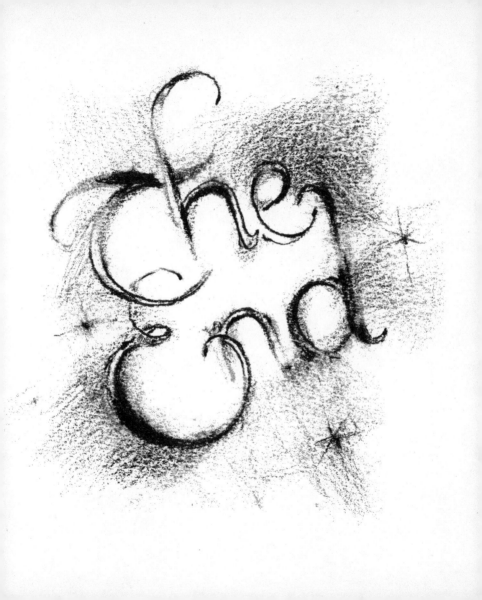

Now I hear my body,
and my body teaches me.

My body teaches me the truth.
The truth is all there is to tell.
Now at the end
I can find the beginning.

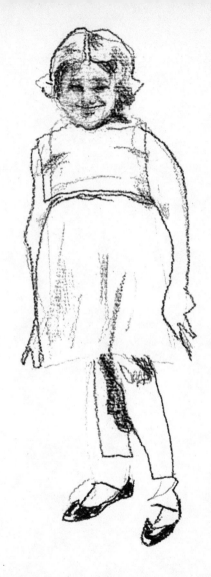

The first day, an everyday day, sways in veils of incense sent by warm molasses cookies . . . I am eight and I come home to no one home or likely to come back soon to these warm molasses cookies. I toss my schoolbooks on the stove, shove two cookies in at once, whinny and get out the milk, drink straight from the carton. Two go in and two go in and two and two and two go in. Sweeter than cookies such freedom to eat them. Devour the missing nourishment.

Thirty gone when thunder struck: Mother would return and see and know. The rest I rearrange like checkers, wipe my mouth across my collar, brush my jumper free of crumbs, run into the living room, jump into the yellow chair, open up my speller there, and spend an hour with a ticking clock.

An hour with a ticking clock is all the guilty need.

Heart beats wild with sugar and remorse.

I hear a car door slam. Her parting laugh. The front door key.

New air comes in.

Her perfumed purse she places on the shelf, hangs her soft coat
deep within the closet, asks would I please hang up mine. I bend
my head into my homework. Yeah, I'll be there. Just a sec. I'll
weep right on your honeycolored ankles.

Fate's made in little moments. The instant that I chose to tell
her, she started up the stairs. Had she won at bridge? I called
instead. She had not, loosening her scarf. Would I call her
please at five? I would. She took the moment with her.
   I sat crosslegged in the yellow chair, teethmarking my pencil
there. No, she didn't see, she couldn't know. Brothers will be
coming home who eat a ton of cookies, so she'll never know.

And not till she'd awaked and cooked and all my
brothers had their seconds did she ask where all the cookies
went. She passed around a plate of ten. If that's what's left of
fifty, then I can't afford to make them anymore. My father
at the table's head said Who. Some brothers said they'd had a
few. But not a lot. I said me too.

My casserole accused me from my plate.

I'll get the table cleared, I said, and grabbed my plate and lurched out through the swinging kitchen door to do the dishes by the ticking clock the ticking clock. Before my water wrinkles smoothed, I'd penciled a confession full as belly and as heart:

i am the liar and the theif. I sware
I'll never eat a cookie in my life again.

I signed it, slipped it underneath my parents' door, and lay awake, soured with the first worst guilt, awaiting the mercy of morning.

but junkies always lie.

I found I was a natural at theft. The Thanksgiving Friday Pie—
a second piece denied me—woke me in the night and issued
orders clear as any parent's voice. I had to follow: Sneak down-
stairs. Avoid the squeak. Into the kitchen. Open the rounded
white door. Strip of light down pajamas shows pie. Slip it out.
Sliver off slivers. Nudge up crust. Suck down custard. Shoot
whip cream in hand. No one's looking. Shoot whip cream in
mouth.

Sound on the stairs.
                              FREEZE.

                                        Slide can down chest, down
thigh, into door. Straighten wax paper. Swing door shut. Slip
out. Creep up steps. Hands like paws on stairs. Toilet flush.

FREEZE.
              Nausea.
                              Crossing enemy lines, the soldier chooses
suicide when there is no escape. Throw
                                        Self
                                                Down
                                                        Stairs
                                                              NOW.

Silence.

      Heart thunder.

      Poised with death on the sixth step.

STEPSTEPstep. Someone going down the hall. Deliverance.
Stair one stair two stair three stair four stair five.
Tiptoe round the corner headfirst into grave
miscalculation—My Father's Arm. Double stun.
Stomach thunder. I'll throw up. Will I throw up
on my father? Help. Help. His hand through my
hair. What is it honey?

Respite. Excuse. Got a splinter in my foot. Got a
needle. In girlscouts we learned how. Shift.
Keep weight off injured foot. I got it out. You
can't even tell where it was. Where is belief?
I got up to get a drink I got it from my floor
I got it in my heelgot a needlegot it out.

Just gray eyes looking. Too dark to see belief if it
is there. Better get to bed now honey. God bless
you. He traces a cross with his thumb on my
forehead. He kisses the cross. Night Dad.

To bedroom home headquarters finish line. Shut the door and shake and shake, sweaty, heavy, leaden with food, but Victorious! Having outsmarted a mom and a dad and me just a kid!

A criminal child. I betrayed my father's trust. My looting and my lies rush to my forehead, burn the cross.

Crime is cold. Shiver. Slip under the covers and shudder. But full. Warmth wombs me. Soon I'm a slow ball rolling toward sleep. On the brink, a jolt of horror splits me like an iron spike. My hand touches cream on my cheek.

Junkies learn to cover tracks.

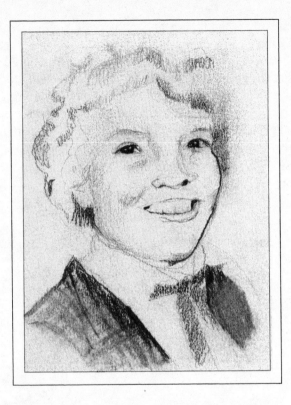

Blessed Bathroom, o Beloved Sanctuary! In your peace and
privacy I eat snuck brownie cuts and bonus oreos, all I palm
from the bridgeclub dish and no one can come in here I am free!

O dearest place to me. Cram the handfuls in and fill the dixie
cup to trickle in the toilet in case somebody's listening. Flush,
then eat the noisy things, straddle toilet seat to check in mirror.
Wipe off clues, wink, slink down, come out zipping up my jeans.
Oh bliss.

Not food, but
my own will
I stole.

Evidence of
treachery grew
daily.

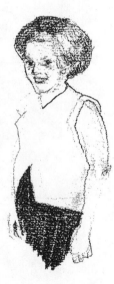

Silver glasses, silver hair, silver moustache, polished German silver voice awhistle with a teakettle "s."

"SSSSSo, ve get our booster shot, eh? Ooopsy daisy, sssit right here. Big girl like you zisss von't hurt. Von two, buckle my shoe, ssree four, shut ze door. All done."

> Well then gimme my sucker.
> "May I have a cherry sucker, please?"

"Shust von little moment. Let'sss come over und ve step on ze scale."

> Had I known I was surrendering, I'd never have stepped aboard.

"Ooooh, tut tut tut, ve are carrying sssome excesss baggich."

> Baggage? My hard-earned victories, my quickwittedness, my own body BAGGAGE?

"Ve must be careful vat ve eat, und not munch ze cookies und ze dumplings now. I tell your Mama ve vatch shust until ve drop zisssss excessssss baggggich."

Lousy bum didn't even give me my sucker. Anger tasted just like hunger. I went home and learned to bake.

Oh, the Bounty and the Benefits of Baking! I first knew and loved you thanks to Santa, who bestowed on me an oven of my own: lightbulb-powered and equipped with tiny spoons and bowls and pans and tiny cake and muffin mixes. And when I'd baked my first jar-top-sized spice cake, I turned it out to cool and drew my thumb across the cake film on the bottom of the pan, wadded it and ate it and was hooked.

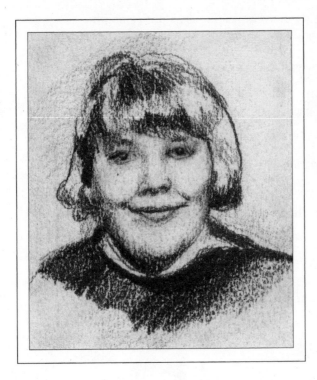

- *Cream* shortening and sugars until smooth.

    take index finger full.

- *Add* eggs and vanilla. Beat till fluffy.

    open chocolate chips. eat handful.

- *Sift* flour, soda, salt together.

    takes too long, just dump it in.

- *Combine* with sugar mixture.

    thick now yes it's sugar clay.

- *Add* chocolate chips and nuts if desired.

    you bet desired oh yes yes big blond dough
    nuggety with nuts and chocolate oh yes
    eat off spoon.

Bake ten to fifteen minutes or until golden brown.

    pop dough in mouth
    look at cookie pictures in
        cookbook

            till . . .

Ding!

               pull 'em out with foldy potholders
               spatulate 'em on the counter
               glassa milk

Let cool.

               one minute
               blow to cool faster
               snugged inside the melty chocolate ouch
               gulp milk
               feel the cookie crispen meeting cold milk
               one after another

Put some on a plate. Just came out of the oven want some?
Yeah! Smelled 'em all through Twilight Zone boy are they great
you make the best ccc's of anyone gotny more?

O Baking! Occupying dismal days, rolling, cutting, punching yeast dough down, slurps off beaters, morsels dollops gobbets mine all mine! And at the end, compliments, thank-yous, genuine attention from the family! Glorious Sanctioned Activity!

My sofa-pillow belly swelled. How powerful I am to change my shape like Zeus! Sugar and hubris sang in my veins until the chants began.

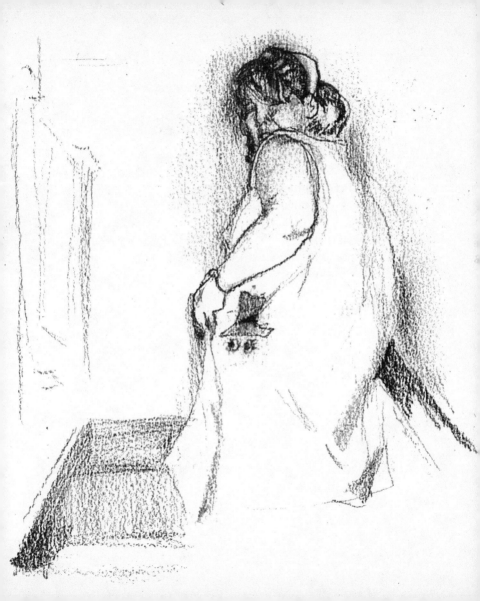

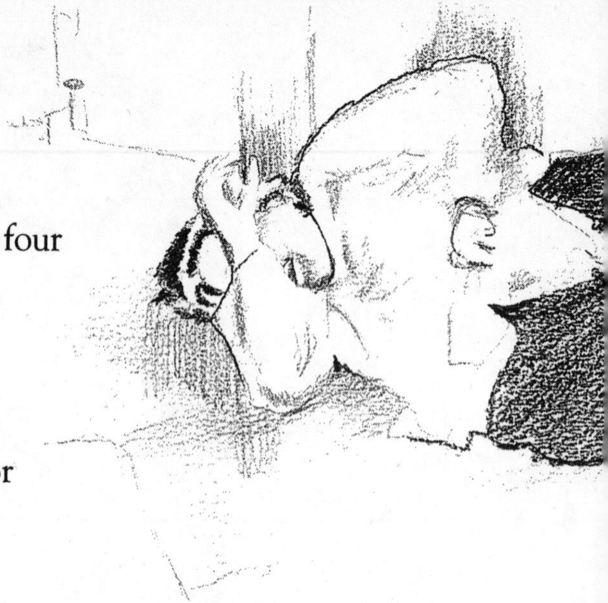

fatty fatty

       two by four

      can't get

through the

     bathroom

        door

    so she

did it

   on the

      floor.

i don't want her
you can have her
she's too fat
for me.

you weigh sixteen tons
and what do you get?
another day older and a-
deeper in sweat.
saint peter doncha call her
cause she'll be late—
she can't fit through
the pearly gates.

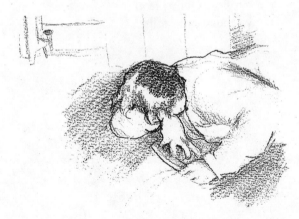

help food save me i'm drowning
get me away from neighbor kids
get me away from me
magic immediate carpet of food
ye hosts of twinkies snowballs carmelcorn
transport me away from friendless saturdays
from rainy afternoons
o my rollover jelly bread
o my sunday sweetrolls

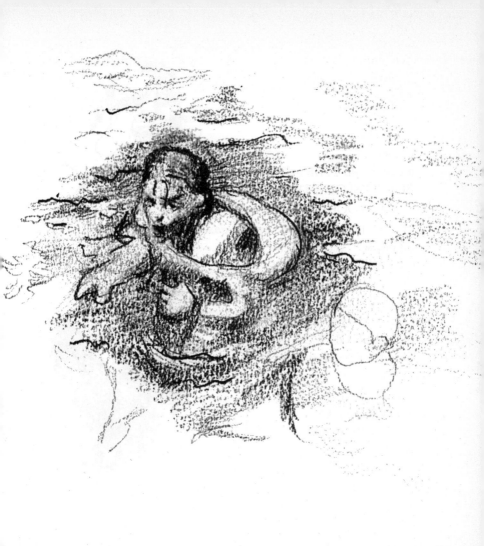

bless me Father for i have sinned it has been one week since
my last confession these are my sins i stole money from
Mother's coat for dairy queen i asked her for other money
i said was for the missions but instead bought milk duds.
and i hate Mrs McCoy.

Honey, there are so many children in Asia who would be
grateful for that Swiss steak. If you don't clean your plate,
no dessert.

>anything for dessert anything. i'd eat the bottom of
>your shoe, Dad.

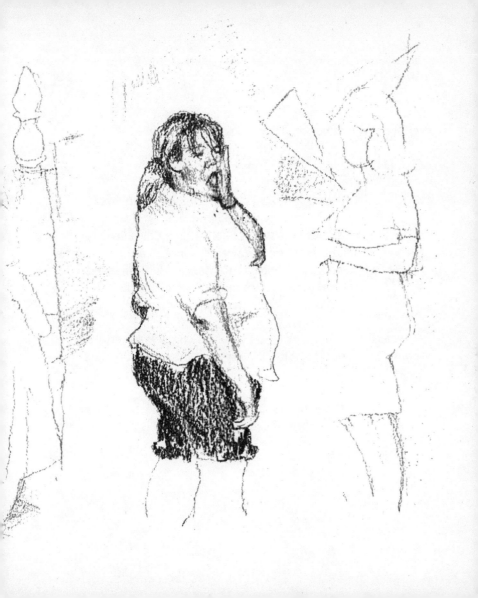

Pants started splitting. Blouses stopped buttoning. Breath slowed.

"Vell, our excesss baggich is now a boxcar. Not good to be chubby. Ve vill be schtrict vid ourself und follow zisss."

REDUCING DIET   typed in purple ink.

> (Alleluia, prodigal child! Ye have sinned, but come unto the fold, be washed pure as snow again! Listen not to the ways of the body that will lead you into temptation and sin, swerve ye not to the right nor to the left, but cleave unto these golden commandments, these proven mathematical standards of eating perfection, and eternal happiness awaits.)

"Ve need sssome insentif. So I give you von dollar for each pound you reduce. SSSirty dollars buys somsssing very nice, my dear."

> Let's see hostess cupcakes are 12¢ so 8 per $1 times 30 is 240 pkgs not bad plus 4¢ times 30 is 24 nickel dairy queens, but to go so long without them . . .

To his silver eyes in silver glasses I agreed; at home with doughnuts in my pockets I spat upon his bribe. Money cannot buy my independence. Looking at his paper through the crumbs, I found the diet's chief delight:

NO cakes candies pies pastries spaghetti bread butter jam.

My fingertip concealed the **NO**.

My eyes ate the words off the page.

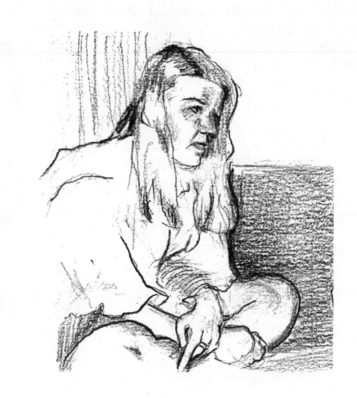

Like most religions, a diet presumes you can't be trusted.
Then you have to prove it. Appetite doubles, stealth triples.

Denied my greatest friend, my Baking, I stole to the bakery,
bought brownies with nickels raked from gritty sofa cracks,
returning at night to demonstrate for family eyes how
scrupulously stringbeans can be measured.

But my Blessed Bathroom then betrayed me to the pink scale beneath her sink. After three weeks of Mother's frown, I devised and reveled in a devilish scheme.

Wednesday next found me lighter by two pounds, though inside the wastebasket inside a bag within a bag were clenched some twenty candy wrappers.

I'd learned to lean my left hand on the sink. Mother beamed, and I pressed harder every week until the inevitable devastating day my sweaty palm slips off the sink. The scale needle jumps like a compass, jabs my mother's heart, sends me flying down a chute of agony:

> i'm sorry mom o please i just wanted you to
> be happy o i'll never do it again i was so bad
> o now you'll never trust me again you'll
> never believe me o dad i don't know why
> i did it you can ground me you can have me
> never eat o you never can forgive me can you

O, my food. The liar that you made of me, the cheat,
the thief.

The punishment for eating
is the punishment of fat.
Subsequently years
and years
of that.

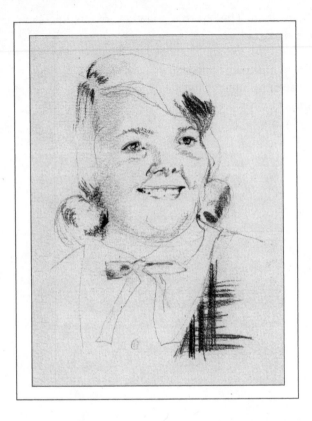

DO NOT READ!

HEY YOU! YES, YOU!
ANYBODY WHO GOT MY KEY AND
UNLOCKED THIS DIARY'S REALLY
GOING TO GET IT!

What's the big idea of prying anyhow, you snoop?
What do I have to do, set
a burglar alarm? Get a fingerprint set?

STAY OUT! MITTS OFF!
GET YOUR PAWS OUT!

HAPPY NEW YEAR

dear diary well a new year is on us and me with a new dear diary it was tragic last year with so many things like Pope John and most of all Pres. Kennedy but this yr will be better i resolve to reduce my weight (in lbs) down to correct weight for my height by end of term and to write each night in you. i love Rick.

dear diary last night i etch-a-sketched that i will not eat anything mom does not ok. just finished "olura" with some pretty ~~sexy~~ "ahem" parts but outside of that a good "house book" (young girls in sinister mansions) which i sure have a knack for picking (accidently) at Bkmobile. You FATTY! REDUCE! i love Rick.

dear diary tomorrow i go on a strict diet so i don't have to in high school kiss pillows instead of ~~boys~~ b's. i love Rick.

dear diary you are my only friend i hate myself i am not normal
i would kill myself to be thin like Karen or even wear a girdle
like Joan K. but mom says no but if i could i would look thin and
Rick would skate with me again o handsomest b in class always
bursting my heart esp when you skated w/ me tho you were just
being polite which we both knew but still

dear diary Lonnie is forever on my mind i don't know if or what
he sees in me i just love handsome him because today in art he
thumped the back of my chair and said how're you doing kid?
i hope he is thinking of me Lonnie Lonnie Lonnie i could write
it forever even though Terry V my best friend likes him too but
i love him more

dear diary i hate lonnie he is a crap wears braces and swares and
Terry V says he makes out with 7th graders crap on him. I WILL
GET THIN!!

dear diary why are people mean Terry V my best friend we were even writing our book Fallen Angel already up to page ten together why would she do what she did tonight which was call me but it was a boy voice i didn't know whose. i took it in the basement by myself my thumpy heart. he said he saw me he said he liked me but just then mom called me to bring the groceries in so would he call me back o please o please. of course he would. at dinner i could hardly eat for once and then it rang and then my torture brother took it and would not get off until at last he did and then it rang it was for me and it was him. i went down to the basement phone he said i was cute and would i go out with him and yesses pulsed all through me but before i spoke i thought how did he know me and where had he seen me and how could he know i make up for my horrible body by my good self and sense of humor wait hey wait who is this anyway giggles laughing in the background this is Terry's birthday and tonite the party i was not invited to i shouted great idea for your party Terry but i wasn't fooled i am not falling for it shut your crap traps all of you and slammed the phone as if it were my heart

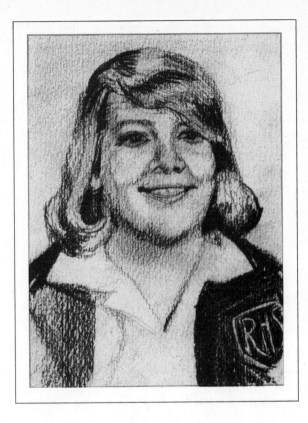

The body reflects what you expect to see. Feeling worthless twists perception like a funhouse mirror:

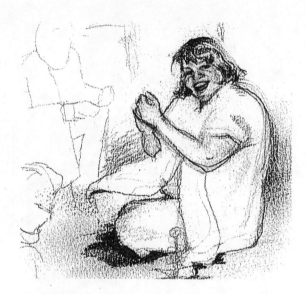

A wimple of fat around my face. Caterpillar-browed scowling
marble eyes. Cheeks thick as kitchen sponges. Pillar of a neck.
Slumping shoulders like a fallen arch. Hammy flopping arms.
Beanbag breasts. Innertube of blubber where the boomerangy
elbows bend, by the monster belly: tub of risen dough. No cunt
visible. Grotesque humps for hips. Whopping ass. Lardy
puckered thighs. Bulging pouches on the kneecaps down the
wide white turkey legs to the fist-ankled weeping feet weeping
feet.

Too fat to cross my legs, too fat to run,
too fat to say body, too fat to say fat.

The slender maid in aspic waits.

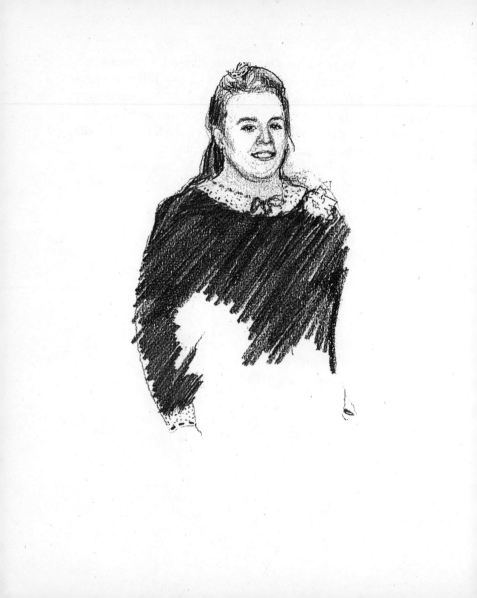

O food, o fat, you robbed me of my youth and dressed me in my middle age. Clothes passed through my life like a funeral procession: black, brown, navy mourned my lifeless body. Scratchy stretchy abominable knits, paisleys in heartbreaking mixtures of colors, jersey dresses feeling like slime dried. The men's shirts, the barrel shorts, the boots that wouldn't pull over my calves.

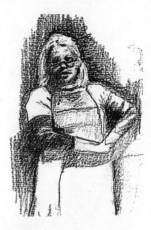

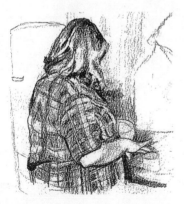

The long successions of dilapidated shoes, sides crushed out, heels rasped off. Beneath the shifts, the muumuus, the tent dresses: longline bras and highwaist girdles, plastic garters cutting in my thighs. Humiliating sound of girdled thighs against each other, zip unzip with every step.

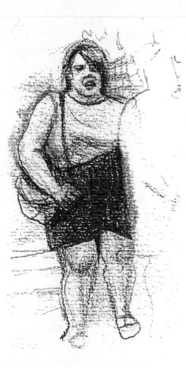

And every zipper
meant suspense—
squish that jiggle
belly in, can the seam
withstand it?
Winter,
sympathetic,
sent me hefty coats,
sweaters
(layers
distract, disguise).
Brutal summer
sweat me like a
plastic raincoat—
on the hottest
day, long pants,
long sleeves;
body never free
of the touch
of itself, dripping
rubber rolls of
rubbing flesh.
I could no longer
stand to hear my
body.

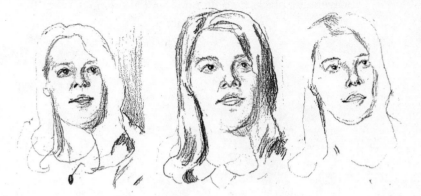

So I grew a self without a body.

A head. A thinker. A smiler. A joker. A listener. A laugher.
A joiner: French Club, News Club, Library, Literary, even
Gym Club. In short, a personality.

Scavenging places fat didn't matter, I also joined
The Drama Club.

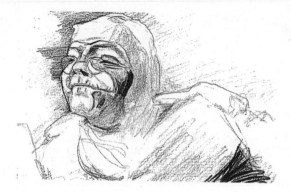

Sweet as warm molasses cookies, the taste of stopping a show.
Howls of laughter and applause at my one line in a one-act in an
instant fed a hundred ancient hungers. My heart knelt at the
moment, saying: I have found the reason I was born.

I made my enemies my audience. No more the victim of their stares, I now commanded them . . . plus wow you get to work with boys which is the best way to get to know them, you know? Not like on dates where everything is nervous. Not that i've been, but a bunch of girls were talking in the can and i think my way's really best where you joke and laugh and find out who's dorky or what but it would be neat just only once a boy's hand at my back guiding me off the hot gym floor at the sock hop for some fresh air but working coat check you find out a lot about guys from their coats, you know? O jeez I'm late for play practice.

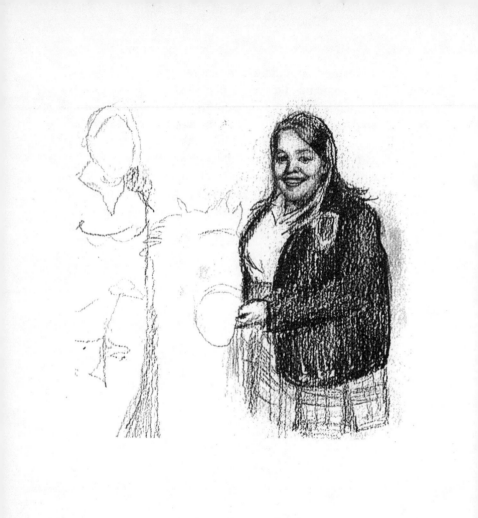

My fat:
my freedom, my distinction, my defense!
What a great sister you made of me!
What a great mother you made of me!
What a scared woman you made of me!

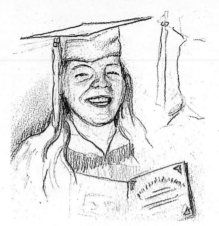

You bullied me through highschool (and I did kiss pillows)
to the miserable midterm midnight dorm and the steady
lighted smile of the vending machine—no human face awake
to shame me—you crammed me full of cupcakes, cherry pies,
candy bars up the stairs and down the hall to my tensor lamp
and pages swimming with text, and bellowed when you saw you
had a rival: my career.

Food was second to rehearsal. Fat was second to my leotard.

To chart my course
I navigated by
the stars:
Hepburn Bernhardt
Duncan Duse Davis.
I read biographies in
junkfood quantities.

And suddenly,
It All Was Clear,
clear as the ting of
a fork on crystal.

IF ONLY
I WOULD LOSE
MY WEIGHT:

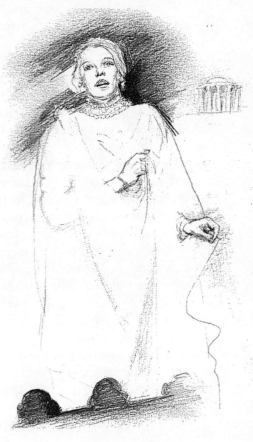

If only I would lose my weight, I will have money, because
then I'll do some modeling because I have a pretty face and
then move to New York and then get in a play and then an
agent sees me and my talent overwhelms him and he gets me in
a brilliant Broadway show and though Kate Hepburn says you
cannot have it all—I would not hope to marry as The Theatre
and marriage do not mix—but such a pack of lovers would line
up outside my dressingroom and send me roses every Broadway
opening which now are coming thick and fast and such intimate dinners with each man so different and I would understand them as no woman ever had and they would love me
more than anyone they'd ever known and would I marry them,
mais non, mais non, avec regret, mon cher petit garçon, The
Theatre is not my life it is my sacrament and it demands I
consecrate my being to it, and with a single smile of mystery
and grace, I would decline, but how the passion would entwine
our hearts and oh the audience wild with clappingtossing
roses showers of flowers billets-doux tears stompthrilling every
night . . . until the evening that I know I am to die . . . and I
bid farewell to Armand and the audience and no one knows
until the curtain call and o my god she died, she really died and
then the outcry and the pouring forth of grief the nation
mourns tonight tonight the world is weeping we are all bereft
thank heavens that we have her down on film but truly there

was nothing like her live upon the stage and such infinities of
wreaths and garlands saturate the air with scent and petal
and like broken branches the black lines of lovers mad with grief
and violently swearing they will make my name and memory
immortal

All of this comes true if I lose weight.

So I'm really going to lose this weight.

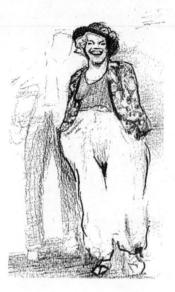

I'm just going to
finish this pound of
M&Ms and these
chocolate-covered
raisins and as soon
as I do, right after
I eat this last package
of oreos and this
peanutbutter ice cream
and the creamfilled
pastry horns,
I'm really going to lose
this weight.

And I really am. I really AM.

Tomorrow I will go on The Strictest Diet There Is.
So strict.

No carbs. Protein. Water. Tab. Cigarettes. Oh, I will be
good so good, I will make these Sacrifices for My Art
and I'm really going to do it tomorrow and be so good
from now on that tonight is the last night I will ever eat
these things so I'll just have this box of Sugar Pops
you know i don't know why people eat vegetables and
oranges when you can put terrific brownies in your
mouth they even taste good frozen so don't wait for
them to thaw i want them now roll up the little
frosting in a ball god why eat broccoli when
these german chocolate cake nuts raisins
bananachipstoffeepopcorncheesecake it's my last
night farewell to all these god
slump over the bed passing out.

Next morning, look in the mirror. Okay, *Ugly*, today is it. The sniper shot stings, but I know I deserve it. Cigarette for breakfast. Hardboiled egg for lunch. Yuck. I'm being good, though, very good. Tab, lots of Tab, Tab with ice, Tab in cans, drink it in class, smoke smoke smoke drink that water keep busy. Plain hamburger, please, no bun. Go to rehearsal. Cigarettes and thoughts of Hepburn when the cast goes for pizza. Smoke guzzle Tab. Got through the first day! I'm really going to do it now! I really AM!

Next day look in the mirror. Fire a few more salvos. Yup. I hate you, body. You're out to get me, you rotten pig, but I'm really gonna fight, and I'm gonna lose this weight and lose it pronto. Stillman says lose 5 lbs a week so I'll be thin Ten Weeks From Today!!!

Smoke smoke growl growl. No, I am in charge here, stomach. Just coffee and Tab for me please. Guzzle.

OH MY GOD I LOST TEN POUNDS!!!

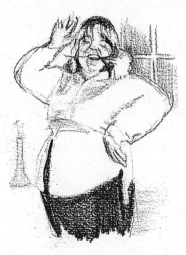

This is great! I really am doing it!! Plain chicken please.
Nibble of skin.

o god. that was bad. oh why did i eat that skin?
i cheated i wrecked my whole diet. you stupid you shit you idiot
you ruined everything! you're off your diet now and for what?
a stupid bite of chicken skin. at least have something decent
for god's sake.

i haven't cheated once except for now. i even got through the
cast party with that beautiful white cake and the oatmeal
cookies. i'll just run really fast to the bakery. may i have half a
dozen, please, or oh I guess a dozen, for a friend, you know, and
a small white cake yes the one with all the roses, oooh, i'll get
them all to myself, and what are these? i'll take a dozen, too, and
now i'll eat these really fast and it won't be so bad so good this
bakery knows its stuff.

i'll get right back on tomorrow. i'll fast all day i promise. mm-
mmchewy oatmeals like i used to bake. i'm so bad why did i gob
that rose. Handful of cake stuff it in. mmmso good who can live
on hardboiled eggs

HOW COULD I EAT ALL THAT

damn this goddamn body. i've got to get out of here, take a walk, think of my career. no one will want me nobody loves me i'm so bad. and i didn't even get any pizza the other night. i'm going right in. one small deluxe pizza please. Cram it in walking down the street piece by piece from the torn box.

GOD I'M SO BAD

jeez i'm so thirsty. oooh a milkshake would cool me down to think. we never got to stop at mcdonald's when i was a kid. i haven't had french fries in so long large fries please and chocolate milk-shake chocolate chocolate marshmallow bunnies at the drug-store hope they're stale they're chewy then. a baby ruth.

GOD I'M SO BAD!! I'M SO BAD!!!

HOW DO YOU EXPECT ANYONE TO LOVE YOU YOU HORRIBLE SOW YOU SLOB YOU TUB OF LARD HOW MANY CHILDREN STARVE WHILE YOU CRAM YOUR GULLET WITH CRAP?

o god let me die

tomorrow i fast

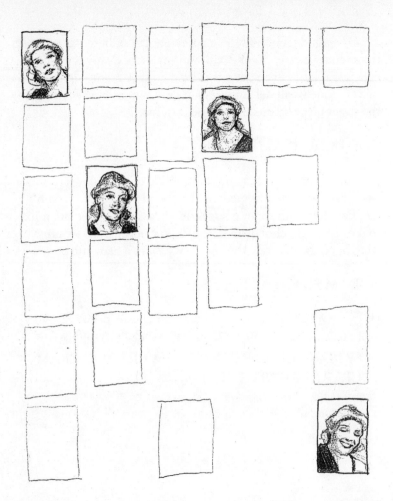

So I lived the litany of diets:

> stillman scarsdale airforce ayds atkins metrecal
> dexatrim grapefruit ten-day wonder two-week fast fast
> fast take it off fast put it on fast. fast.

The punishment for eating is the punishment of fat,
and dieting's the punishment for that.

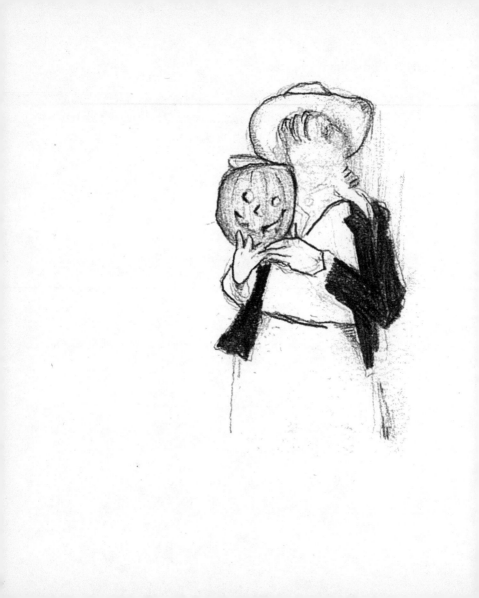

To diet is to battle in a mirror. There's the enemy. The sight inspires the hatred that's the pumping heart of war that drums in every vein until the beating is a trance and the trance is dedication to supreme annihilation of the execrable evil of the enemy out there. The beating's beating: beat her back and up and down, the drum drills killing, when the question comes the answer springs Yes Sir! Ready Sir!

Charge the Hill and Take it, Sir!

YES AT ANY COST SIR!!!

CHAAAAAAAAAAAAAAAAAAAARGE!

alone on the field. who is my ally? my body is my enemy. i multiply my enemy myself. choke with recognition. like every human war, a civil war.

The Goal, Sir? Control, Sir. Club the self into submission, Sir. Eliminate the chance of further treason, Sir.

The mirror is the battleground, so tactics are reversed. To win is to lose, to lose: to gain. A steep hill, not to seize, but to descend not running. A soundless war: no bugle, no attack, no flag. A war of ration cards, of sober choice; to passively resist the brutal urges of the enemy i mistook for the heroine.
o my breaking blue heart.

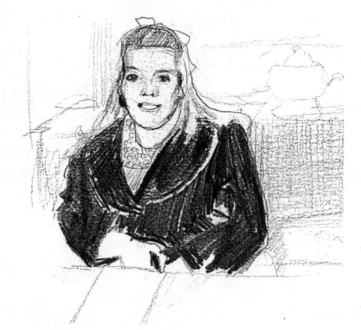

Awareness slips like a spy through the lines. An echo of a whisper: trust is the only victory, and can't be forced.

I'm too fearful to believe.

Cheated of a fair fight, cheated of my food, I cheated until cheating didn't taste good anymore. Desperation and my sister's losing sixty pounds drove me to a weightloss group.

Now, mostly the way I looked at groups was as something from which to distinguish myself: A family's to get their attention. A class is to be teacher's pet. A team is to be the best player. A party is to be the life of. A crowd is to stand out in. A cast: to be the star. A generation: an outstanding member. All humans of all time: unique.

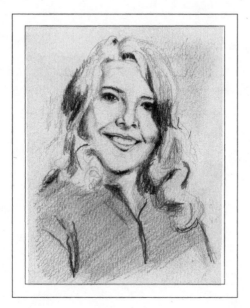

This was, of course, American of me. In the land of assassins and stars, we work so hard to make ourselves alone. And everyone else's awareness of us is always more important than our own.

Two ways to stand out in a group: succeed brilliantly, miserably flop. I joined one and did both.

At my weightloss group
I learned a score of
brandnew habits:
Eat three nourishing
meals. Keep track
of what is eaten. Plan.
Prepare. Put fork down
between bites.
Don't shop hungry.
Set a pretty table.
Don't eat standing up.
Never, never skip a meal.

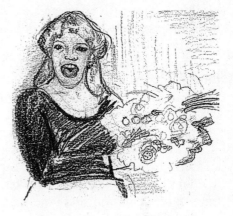

In six months I lost forty pounds.

O Bliss! I wasn't hungry. I was losing weight. People said how great I looked, and at last I knew that I was Truly Good, for all throughout Thanksgiving and my birthday and my Christmas and my every ounce of forty pounds, I never, never cheated once.

Pride goeth.

I gave my landlord notice, loaded everything into a U-Haul, and hit the highway high on me and my accomplishment, paused midcarrot as I passed the Statue of Liberty standing like an Oscar in the sunset . . .

I drank deep my dream come true, through my first audition, through my first leading role, through my good reviews, and yes! an agent came to see the show! And yes! He likes my work! "But if you're serious about the theater, you'd better lose that weight."

The next day for the first time, I skipped lunch.

I was hungry when I reached the Greek restaurant at 49th and 8th where I went for dinner by myself, and there, God bless it, on my table the waiter put a basket of the freshest and most fragrant bread in town, and I was lost.

I had six months' denial to make up for, and I spent three years at it. I dangled "tomorrow" in front of myself and spun my sugar gyroscope again. My food, my fat, my old familiar faults. My comfortable pendulum: obsession and oblivion. Poe's pendulum.

Then the inevitable night when it swung low enough to slice and nearly bleed me dead.

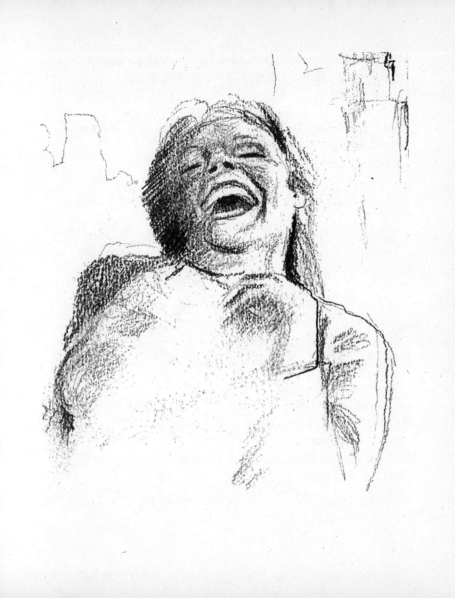

It started off like any night alone. Dinner and the news.
jeez so much i should do: write letters, read, study,
become perfect.

Pace. Still hungry. Pull open cupboard. Rock back and forth.
Take down cereal. Unroll bag. Grab handful.
The Bitch Within awakens.

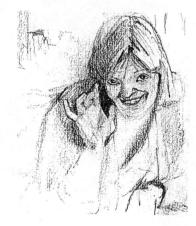

Dry cereal, my dear?
We don't even put it in a bowl like humans anymore?
        lemme alone.
Swing open freezer. In frost mist, chew frozen bread.

How revolting! Can't even wait for it to thaw, you flopbellied
bottomless pit!

        shut up you shit

I'm only the observer, dearie. You're the one who's shoveling
it in.

        lemme alone. i'll get thin, you'll see.

Bet you twenty pounds of Sara Lee.

        i'll show you. i'll buy the scarsdale book right now, do
        two weeks, drop twenty and go back to WW.

Fat chance.

        i'm leaving.

I know where you're going and what for. Can't fool me.

Coat on. Out door. Down elevator. Half hour later back at the
apartment.

Certainly took our sweet time. Make some extra stops, Pudge?

        shut up i'm reading my diet book, see?

Indeed I do, and I must say it was sheer inspiration to buy
doughnuts, too. Greasy fingers turn pages better.

        look, this is my last night, so i'm entitled.

Oh, forgive me. With your sterling record, heaven forbid I should doubt your commitment. What else have we in our little diet bag? Oooh. Isn't this cute? Mother Earth News and a bag of granola! How sixties. And Vogue! I knew a gorgeous creature like you had to have her beauty secrets! Tell me, though. How do you handle the obvious futility?

shut up shut up lemme read

Rumpbody, even I know the damn thing by heart. Poultry fish fruit veg—how much cash will you keep shelling out to read the same crap over and over?

Shut up! Doughnut doughnut doughnut. Granola granola granola.

Remember when your teeth were so sugar-rotted it hurt to chew granola? When the dentist found twenty-two cavities? Cheer up. You'll have to quit eating when all your teeth fall out.

LET ME OUT!

Back outdoors on automatic pilot. No concept of the weather or the time, although it's midnight blowing snow. Buy surefire foods. Chocolate chip cookie box torn and minus three before the deli door rings my exit. Stuff the chocolate pinwheels in going up the elevator. C'mon you babies, work for me tonight. C'mon.

God they're not working.
Unlock the door. Push into apartment.
Work goddammit cookies!

Pendulum night. No escape.

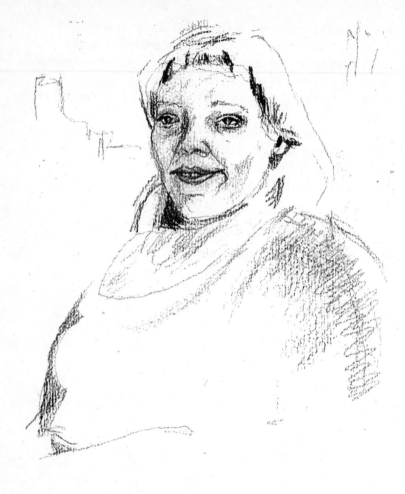

The squalor of the binged apartment struck me like a sandbag. The grease-stained grocery bags. The shredded packaging. The crumpled cellophane. The grubby twisted cardboard. The sugar dirt. The opened emptied cans. Crusts and crumbs and lumps of food strewn about like showered lava. o my god

Well you deserve this shitty sty, you pig. You're not worth cleaning up for and why bother? You'll only stink it up again tomorrow. Besides, I think you like to wallow in it. That's where they'll find you dead like Mama Cass, choked on some gigantic mass of food, and they'll come in this place you've fouled and find you slumped over the garbage and bury you in a piano crate!

Ramming chocolate cookies in. why don't they work they don't taste good o help me help me why am i doing this i want this out of me there is no pleasure i despise food get it out get it out

Where are you going?
            o my blessed bathroom sanctuary peace place

You're not really going to—
            get out of me i hate you i hate you

You DISGUSTING EXCREMENT! Everyone you know should see you right here now with your fucking finger down your fucking throat! O MY GOD!

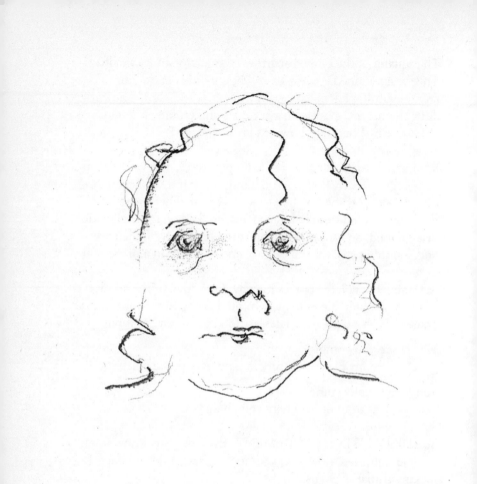

The gagging agony. Tears sweat vomit vortex down the toilet.
Head hung. Dripping face. Tremble throbbing throat. Bitter
bitter mouth. Shaken breath. A moment . . . Lift my head.
The red-rimmed mirrored eye beholds an utterly degraded
human being.

Quaking knees release. Hot red cheek on icy porcelain.
Weep weep. Weep weep. Amnesia of sleep.
    Awakening. Remembering. No stitch of dignity to drape it
now, i see my ugly bulging soul exposed in morning light.
A beached whale, scarce breathing, longing for death.

i must go out. No response. Even the bitch has fled.
Step into a sheet of skirt, wind me in a billow shirt, button up
my binding coat, slud the numb streets up and down, a blank . . .
adrift the blank of fallen snow.
    Daylight empties into night, sound to still, me to nothing.
    Void upon a vacant chair. So nothing now I cannot feel to
fear the darkness or the silence.

Then, of course, occurs the ordinary miracle:

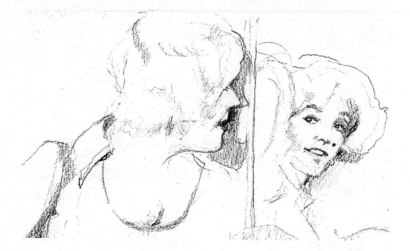

from nothing, something.

The blades of my despair that plowed me through had left me open as a furrow field where fell that night new seed, seed planted in the dark, to light pulled upward strong as gravity, and as eclipsing and elapsing time proves dawn the blossom of the night, one day awareness spoke again:

You're going to be all right.
>   Who goes there? Friend or foe? i am a single crazy
>   soldier in a foxhole.

You know me. Be gentle with yourself.
>   i hate myself. i hate my life.

Hate's just hurt turned. You don't pull at other people's wounds. Let yours heal. There was a reason for the other night.
>   Yeah. i'm scum.

Back since warm molasses cookies, you've tried to gorge away the knowledge that an excess is as painful as a need. The other night you rammed the pain beside its cause. You're trying to connect them. You're trying to get yourself to stop.
>   i'm trying not to do this anymore.
>   My muscles start to quake. My breath begins again.

You'll find a way to heal.

The warm voice bandages my heart.

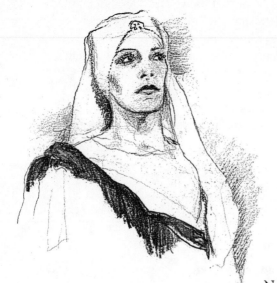

Next day I found
myself outside a
bookstore in
the Village clutching a book that looked
at fat through feminism.

Well, we are scraping the bottom of the barrel, aren't we, Barrelbottom? Buying anybody's radical crap to put the blame anywhere but on your own flabby will. I'm amazed you even have the gall to stand on a public street with decent human beings after your revolting foray into Ancient Rome the other night.

No response. I was reading.

I had an almost chemical reaction to the book.
The catalyst: overeating implies a desire to be fat.
        Impossible! My thoroughest desire is to be thin.
The enzymes: then why have you never been?
        I'm weak.
Nobody weak can fast for two weeks. Nobody weak stays fat in a culture despising it. It costs too much. But it must benefit you.

        How?

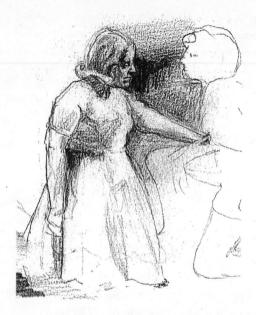

Thoughts I'd been too scared to think.
Amino answers formed:

You bet I'm fat. At least I'm big. I take up space. You can't ignore me or confuse me with some empty-headed petty thing obsessed with her appearance, diddle-brained subservient ridiculous and catty, can't make up her mind. Not me. See here my intellect is nimble as a gymnast, cuts a figure like a Beardsley nymph, like a ballet star, and it goes the body one better, for it shan't break down with age but be refined enriched illuminated through the course of time.

Answers linked together into reasons, rushed like proteins to my starving psychic tissues:

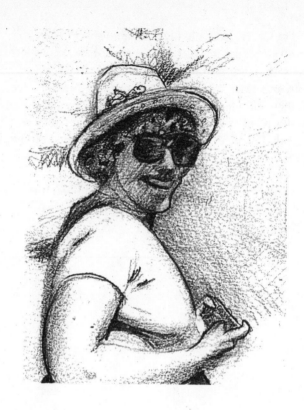

Sometimes I am a fat woman to be noticed. Sometimes I am a fat woman to be ignored. Sometimes I am a fat woman to defy the movies and the magazines. Sometimes I am a fat woman to say no to men without creating injury or rage. Sometimes I am a fat woman because addiction is convenient and perfection easy in the mind. Sometimes I am a fat woman since then I have a foot between the sexes.

A lot lives in a heart.

> **Wmn** int'std in forming self-
> help grp based on Fat &
> Feminism, call Gail 555-1979.

Out of a Westside free newspaper, nine strangers met one
Wednesday night, and all of us afraid. And all arranged to meet
next week, and not one thought she would return (the issues
were too intimate to share). And five showed up the Wednesday
next: Willa and Gail and Dulcey and Ellen and me.

Once a week we sat in a circle and talked, made up exercises,
drew pictures, shared photographs, traumas, and questions.

What scares us about being thin? What do we think when we
see a thin well-dressed woman? What is our reaction when we
see a fat woman? How do we feel about our bodies? What is our
best feature? How do we feel about clothes? How would we dress
thin? What messages did our mothers give us about our bodies?
Our weight? The way we dress? When were we thinnest? Why?
How do we feel about our sexual selves? How do men respond to
us? How do we respond to them? What messages do we think
our fat is sending? To whom? How can we be thin and still be
ourselves?

Our goal was not to lose weight but to break emotional
addiction to food. The book said do not diet, and we didn't.

O first freedom since my excess-baggage days: not to diet or to binge, but to eat when I'm hungry what I'm hungry for! To start to listen to the body, which will regulate itself and tell me when it's full. The feeling of not dieting equal to the sensation of liberty when a college movement teacher turned off all the lights, put music on, and told our class, "Dance however you will. No one can see." My body wept and leapt and danced its story for the first time.

A group in harmony is like a temporary body, members nourishing each other, furthering a higher purpose and awareness. As a friend says, "You have to do it yourself, but you don't have to do it alone."

How less alone I was, not yet *in* my body, but feeling it at my side; hearing from time to time its soft suggestions: enjoy this food now, give me sleep, now I want fresh air.

These were teaspoons of love through the day—strange sweet substance when you're used to hardtack.

Feel the years of coiled defense relaxing, lay the weapons down, lift martial law, declare the truce.

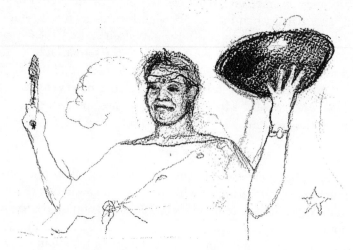

Groups are to be a part of, not apart from.

After six months, as one we sensed that it was time to let each other go. We bid farewell at dinner at a fancy restaurant—the first and last meal that we ever shared.

Then I ambushed myself in the mirror again.

I accept what I feel, but not how I look.
Culture had me on its hook.

Back to WW. Stumble. Back again, stumble again, back again,
stumble again, stop.
why do i poison my career? i've wanted it as fiercely as wanting
to be thin. A bell rang. Perhaps I didn't want to act.
(A thought as revolutionary as Copernicus.)

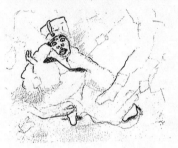

A Theatre Life. I can't control if I work, when I work, where
I work, on what I work, how long I work, with whom I work.

I only control my own moments on stage, and these I repeat every night after night. Mais non, mais non, avec regret. Beloved Rose, I scoop you up and fling you to my past.

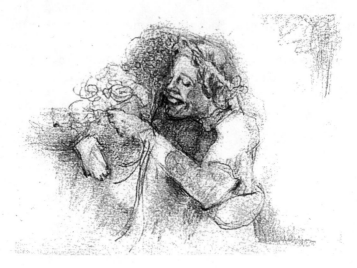

During those stumbles, the man who, though we'd had our rocky times, fulfilled the fatgirl fantasy (loved me for myself alone and not my yellow hair) gently said he worried for my health.

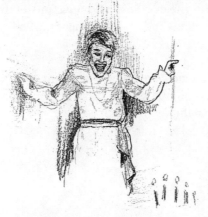

Back to WW once and for all. Nourish swim dance. 50 lbs gone. For once it dawned on me that I could gain it back. Onto the cereal and pasta shelf, I taped up pictures of my old fat self.

Minus 65, I listed changes:
I eat more slowly. I love to move, so there Mrs Stinking McCoy.
I keep flour and sugar without mixing cookies. I rarely binge,
and I can stop in the middle of one. I can maintain my weight
even in foreign lands and . . . now I hear my body and my body
teaches me.

My body teaches me democracy. My womb does not despise my
feet. My kidneys do not wish to be my fingers. Lung, stomach,
none smarter. Brain, marrow, none better. Eye no more deserv-
ing than anyone else. From each to each's need: food, rest, work.
We have to be ourselves to enjoy ourselves.

Yes! It's a superb catch by Number 23, the running back, and she's running with it—look at her go! She's on the sixty, the fifty, the forty-yard line—what a magnificent runner! She's on the twenty—the ten— What?!! What's she doing?! I can't believe my eyes! Folks, this reporter has never seen anything like it! After a spectacular seventy-five-yard run, 23 has stopped running ten yards from the goalpost! Oh! She's dropping the ball—she's walking back to the other goal! Oh—no wait—she's turning around—she's not picking up the ball, though—she's rolling it around with her foot!! This is incredible!! Run, you idiot!! I'm sorry, folks, it's just that when you've seen such a tremen—What a shame—she's just walking back and forth—ten bloomin' yards from the goalpost! I don't understand it, folks—just heartbreaking.

The running back walked back and forth in front of the goalpost for nine months.

> i am a saboteur and i am subtle, dark,
> precise. i do my work in silence, snip,
> clog, spoil. bit of bread by bit of meat,
> i keep me from my goal.

Awareness probes.

What is your goal? Numbers on a scale or dress?
   How can I settle for less?

Where'd you get that goal?
   Everybody knows. Magazines and stores and shows.
   Wish we lived in Rubens's time, but these are
   different days.

Anybody profit from your not being at goal weight?
   I'm not interested in this line of thought.

Dissatisfaction's a vacuum industries suck money through.
   What difference does that make?

Are you happy trying to reach a certain weight?
   No, but what choice do I have?

You can choose a goal that makes you happy on the way.
   Forget it. I'm not giving up.

Certain days, my body is a haunted house, secreting shadows till i cannot tell the darkness from myself. Then a caress.

        Who's there?

Touches urging all along me.

        Stop. Who is it?

Silence shivers with a whisper: *yes you miss us. let us in again.*

        Who are you?

your oldest lovers lining up to love you once again.

And caresses and caresses and incessant whispering insisting: *let us back. you love us and you need us.*

Stroking, stroking soft as drugs.

        Let me see you.

Feel delicious yielding. Yes   about to loosen from my lips.

NO like lightning crashes. By flash I glimpse the grotesque faces—ghosts of guilt and fear and shame and anger packaged into pounds, surrounding, begging me.

        NO YOU ARE DEAD.

Laughter. Loathing moans smoke through my thighs. Rusted passion rattles in my belly. Raw wails swell my hips. *!let us back!* Stroking goes to striking. They pound hot fury into freezing shrieks. *!the passion was too great you never can be free! !just see!*

Wave of nausea bobs a buried body up. Perpendicular cadaver of my loathed old self confronts me like a murdered king demanding restitution. Some nights the king has force to make me yield to his ghost legions fouling my house. Some nights I force myself to stare into his rotting face till daybreak.

I tell myself he stinks because he's dead. The face is hideous because it's decomposing, it's falling apart, it's going away. These pounds, these thoughts are dead, they have no power. My imagination animating's all it is. Daybreak always comes. The vision is less vivid every time.

Still, i am a saboteur and i am subtle,
dark, precise. i do my work in silence,
snip, clog, spoil. bit of bread by bit of
meat, i keep me from my goal.

Could I just forgive myself? Could I face my fear?
Could I change my goal?
The saboteur is shifting to the side. My body's moving in.

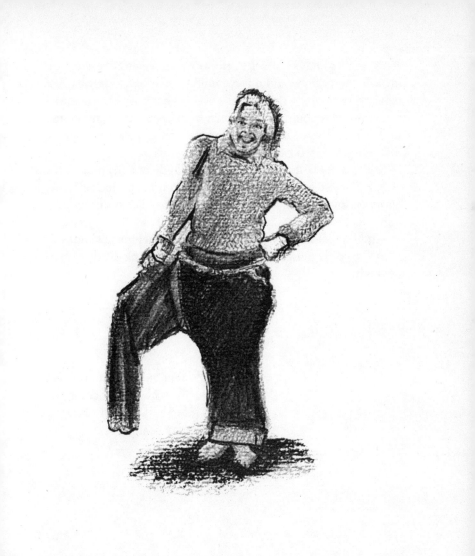

And yet this body's scary. I've never had a skeleton or edges to myself before. Bone and muscle hold no mystery, so frank beneath my sagging skin: some sorrow is coming, sad shadows, some sorrow is coming. I've grown limits. My body is no more no less than these same sad curves seen on a million women. Such disappointed bones say that life is toil.

Still got my belly dough, my good ol' pile of belly dough, the grand ol' waist-wide thighs, but no, my round familiar self is— disappearing, leaving a bony woman in an old skin suit that hangs embarrassing as fallen pants.

And I'm colder now, my padding gone. Feel my jawbone. Spot the cordy muscles in my neck. At last I link death with my body.

so i am a saboteur and i am subtle, dark, precise. i do my work in silence, snip, clog, spoil. bit of bread by bit of meat, i keep me from my goal.

I see death in the mirror. Love wells up. I no longer long for it. But how do I accept it, spelled along my limbs so clearly?

Then I hear my body, and my body teaches me.

My body teaches me my need and my enough. My body teaches my enough of life is death, and that the way to die is sitting down, or turning, or to bend, or leaning, or upright with a gesture, or facedown, or to curl. To be feared no more than sitting after standing, stretching after sleep. Death is but a change of posture.

My body changes all the time, with moon, with age, with weather. Change is the respiration of existence.

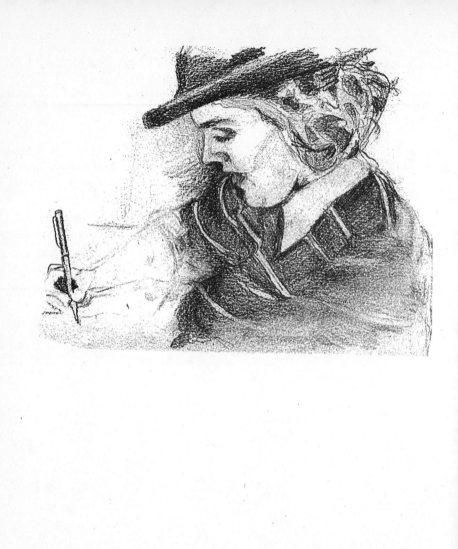

20 May, 11:45 P.M. Session with Inner Analyst.

You're quite troubled. Tell about your week.
>Concisely: shit. Back from Seattle. Didn't diet, but in control on trip. 3 lb gain at WW. Furious. Did not deserve. Went out and ate food worth a 3 lb gain. Stupid. Probably only had gained a pound and a half since was preperiod.
>Back on program. Struggled. 3 days legal. Had dinner guests tonight. Face depressing weigh-in tomorrow. Week is shot. Overate, not even wanting to.
>Why so stupid? Counterproductive? Not fear of success. Lost 75 lbs. I like my success.
>Not self-hatred. Like me more than ever.
>WHY AM I FAILING AND FAILING? WHY CAN'T I FINISH THIS OFF?

Say you were an architect. Your goal: to build yourself a house. Would you blueprint rooms you didn't want to build?
Would you draw up lists of fixtures you dislike and catalogue each tool that wouldn't help you on the job? Page through your portfolio instead. Look at your success, and then we'll talk about the house.

I wear short hair for
the first time.
I don't hate cameras,
mirrors, plate glass.
I bare my collarbone,
my shoulders,
the sluices of muscle
in my upper arm,
wear T-shirts easy as
a tomboy, curvy
dresses happy
as a prom girl.

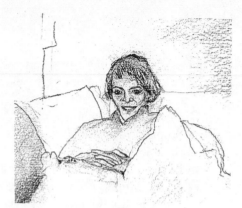

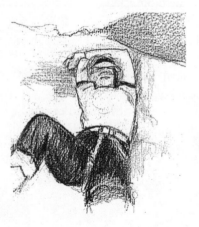

A waist, by god, to pass
 elbows through, to tuck
shirts into, to belt. I, who was
not delicate, have delicacy
now in wrist and hand.
I'm unafraid to show my hips
in jeans, to buckle up
a seatbelt.

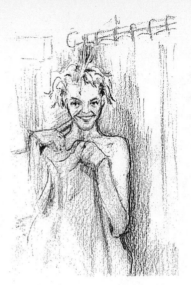

To be deliciously at ease in lingerie, to be naked and joyful to be naked, to feel light as childhood, to take up less space and feel far more entitled to it.

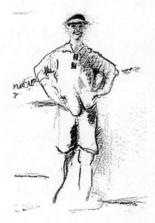

Pantyhose fit. I don't feel sick in clothing stores. I wear shorts. Kneesox stay up on legs I like to see and move, and I can cross them, too. I'm stronger and I'm swifter and my gestures and my postures don't apologize.

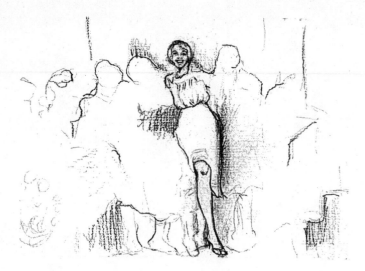

High heels don't crush my happy dancy feet dancy feet.

Good. Go deeper. What have you learned?
> I'm more aware, for one thing. I'm kinder to myself.
> I'm on my side. And even though I can't control my
> emotions, I can control my behavior.

"Control" sounds like you still think you can't trust yourself.
> Well, under certain circumstances . . .

Like what?

        I screw up when I think of weighing in!

You don't ever have to weigh yourself again.

        What?! But but I haven't reached goal weight.

Those are someone else's house plans. You have the right to build the place you want to live. Use your imagination. What's your dream house?

        I'm sick of defending myself. I want to scrap the missiles pointed at my heart and use my energy for other things. I want to feel good and look good without regimentation. But I'm scared.

WELL, say good-bye to all those fears for good, because we've got something right back here (*shakes glitter curtain*) that will solve your eating problems FOREVER! That's right! Throw away your diet books! (*toss*) NEVER count calories again! (*rip*) Get rid of that bathroom scale!! (*sledgehammer*) This incredible EATING MONITOR tells you when to eat! (*taps watch*) What to eat! (*waves menus*) And an automatic signal goes off EXACTLY when you've had enough! (*ding*) No measuring, and no guesswork!! All you do is listen—it does ALL THE REST! It's amazing! Breakfast! Lunch! Dinner! (*flying silverware*) Even tracks those pesky snacks! (*burst of cheez curls*) PLUS THERE'S MORE!! Needs no electricity! And it's fully portable!! No one will ever know you're using it!! Why *(tugs lapels)*, I'm using one right now! *(pulls down map)* Scientists all over the world call it a MIRACLE, and you will too!!! Best of all, it comes with a LIFETIME GUARANTEE!! What would you pay for this INCREDIBLE VALUE?? *(flings bills)* $1,000? $100? $29.95? Tell ya what I'm gonna do. I'm gonna let you have this fully automatic

MIRACLE EATING MONITOR

absolutely FREE
at no cost to you, the lucky user!

(yanks curtain back to reveal mirror)

My body. My human body.

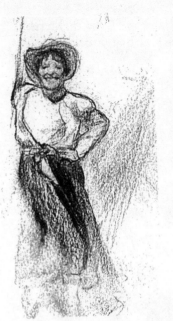

Next day I checked in with the metal warden one last time and floated through the swinging prison door.

I read books which encouraged me to hear my inner voice above the din of culture. I encountered the idea that our beliefs create reality, as the architect the house, and I began to try it out.

I swallowed cups of love.

But then we moved into a life upstate, and like a frightened child creeping back to a big secure armchair, I took my heavy body once again.

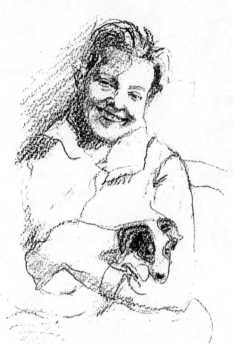

It is a human thing to pick an easy pain above a pleasure that's an effort.

I was gentler with myself this time.

Do you think there might be reasons other than weight that made you feel so bad about yourself throughout your life?
        Maybe.
What was the fat little girl after?
        Someone to listen, for one thing.

Psychotherapy? You chicken shit! Who do you think you are? Olivia de Haviland in *Snake Pit?* What good is talking about it going to do? You've talked about it your whole damn life. You just keep making excuses, you coward, you spineless pile of blubber.

One burning hot July, reeling with the venom of The Bitch Within, I came to understand there's such a thing as toxic thought. For once, instead of changing food or eating habits, I chose to change my thoughts. And since The Bitch Within was formidable, I knew I needed help. I found someone wise, who listened with love.

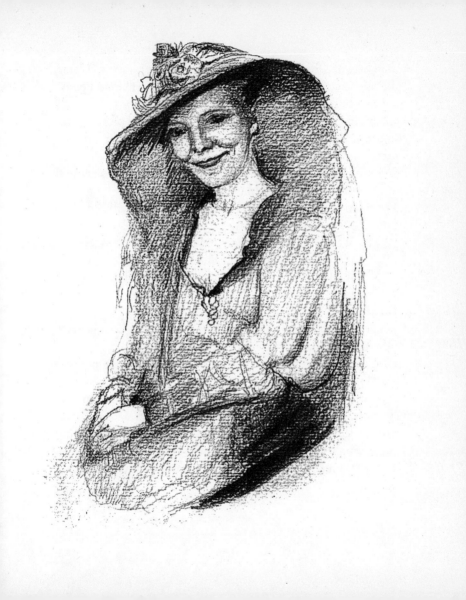

A daughter of Original Sin, I'd always thought myself to blame, and I was unaware, until I told my stories, of the fear and pain that brought me there.

I learned about my parents' cruelty, and of their sorry ignorance, and what, in the context of their culture and their church, they meant as love. But that's another story.

I saw why I had done what I had done, and how this made the who of me. I then let go of blame.

I ferreted out beliefs I'd held unknowingly and without question:

> It's wrong and vain to care for your appearance.
> How can you be happy when so many people suffer?
> If you are unhappy enough, maybe you'll deserve joy.

I then let go of what's to be deserved.

I shook hands with the mirror. I embraced it. It became a loving friend. I then let go of fifty pounds.

Now I try to bathe in love, to drink it in, to saturate my pores. My goal is a complete transfusion.

And when I retell my tale, instead of seeing failed attempts at weightloss, I see stages in an education of myself.

First grade: learning how to eat. Sixth grade: learning loving exercise. High school: learning to direct behavior. College: learning to direct beliefs. My Ph.D.: learning to love myself.

I wish I could have learned them in reverse. Loving of the self comes first. Without it, there's no body, no relationship, no work, no wealth, no pleasure, no philosophy that will fulfill.

And when it is abundant, coursing through the veins, the body, mind, and soul are all transformed. It radiates at once to other bodies, shimmers in the eyes, the hands, the voice, the actions.

Behold! it cries. See the beauty of the fat girl! See the grace and vigor of her curving body! Celebrate the glory of big women! See them in the sauna and the steamroom, firm and stately presences, heroic as Picasso found them, lush in their repose as Renoir saw, majestic as the Renaissance.

And again Behold! it cries. All body shapes, sizes, colors, ages, and abilities are beautiful! See these dignities! Each holds awareness, suffering, hope, and effort in its heart, and every eye reveals this, and every body teaches us.

I gather up the cookie-bloated child, the aching-hearted teen, the wounded Bitch Within, and thank them all for teaching me. I give them love. I let them go.

Who takes their place?

A body supple with beliefs:
   Now I love my body and my body loves me back. I love this face, these arms, these breasts, this waist, these hips, these thighs, these legs as they are now. For if I lose another five or seven pounds, my cheeks go gaunt, my breasts both disappear, and these thighs and hips are still these thighs and hips. And so I love them now.
   I am graduated. I am trim and fit and secure in it. I choose a healthy form. I trust myself. I am in my prime. I am who I want to be. I am The Queen of Me Land. I am a living happy ending. And now I hear my body, and my body teaches me.

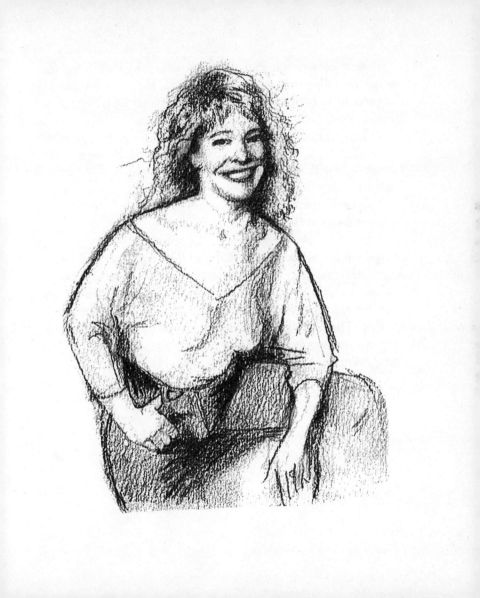

My body teaches me that all things pass. And if all things in life are always passing, it means that Life Is Flow. We are flowing through our lives like blood, like air through lungs, like sight through eyes.

And the gift of flow is that it can be changed at any point, by the smallest rock, the biggest boulder. Belief and choice and effort are the rocks and boulders which change the flow of life at any point.

My body teaches me my soul. My soul seeks what my body proves: balance and perfection. Nothing is more perfect than the whole cloth of my breath unwound without a rip since birth, nor more balanced than even at two hundred pounds, my body walking. The levels in my blood, my steady pumping heart, my eyes' resolve to gray, my left and right. Biology is symmetry is me. And humans are one body on the body of the earth.

And this, our body teaches us, is peace. Peace all the time like space is everywhere. All the time like space this shapeless peace is changing. As incorruptible, as indestructible as space, this peace is always as complete, as even and as ancient, as eternal, as embracing, and as obvious as space.

This our body teaches: All pains are growing pains. All pains are flowing pains. Pain's not a random thing. We hurt to be aware.

Awareness is Omnipotent.
Nothing in the universe can stop Her.
Awareness is Omnipotent.
Everything leads to Her.
Nothing is beneath Her.
Nothing is beyond Her.
Nothing but Herself.

Books That Assisted Me

Orbach, Susie. *Fat Is a Feminist Issue*. New York: Berkley Pub, 1982.

Roberts, Jane. *The Nature of Personal Reality: A Seth Book*. Englewood Cliffs, NJ: Prentice-Hall, 1976.

Roberts, Jane. *Seth Speaks: The Eternal Validity of the Soul*. New York: Bantam Books, 1985.

Suzuki, Shunryu. *Zen Mind, Beginner's Mind*. (Trudy Dixon, ed.) New York: Weatherhill, 1970.

Wolf, Naomi. *The Beauty Myth: How Images of Beauty Are Against Women*. New York: Morrow, 1991.

Acknowledgments

This book has reached your hands by virtue of the love, support, and talents of many people and with the assistance of several organizations.

My first thanks go to Eleanor Torrey West and her artists' colony on Ossabaw Island, where I began this book, and to Carol Burdick and the colony at Alfred University, where I continued it.

Jorie MacKinnon, Vay David, and Jenna Zark have my love for the magnificent incubator called The Bridge Club.

I am most grateful to the Garrison Art Center, Garrison, New York, and Poets and Writers in New York City for the space, money, and encouragement to bring my work to the public.

Thanks to the Church of Saint Philip's, Garrison, New York, Vassar College, Marist College, Stonehill Theatre, Beekman General Store, and the Gathering at Bigfork for inviting me to perform and refine this piece.

I warmly acknowledge the efforts and encouragement of Jeannine Edmunds, Laura Blake, Phoebe Kaylor, Brydon Fitzgerald, and Doug Cole and the lifelong support of Robin O'Brien.

For opening hearts and doors for me, particular thanks go to Linda Ford Blaikie and Jean Marzollo. I also acknowledge the inspiring work of Jane Roberts and Robert Butts.

Molly Friedrich, thanks for chancing it; Amy Hertz, I so appreciate your talents and our resonance. Special thanks to Jaime Robles and the staff at HarperSan Francisco for their excellent work.

Deep bows of gratitude to the Women's Circle for the magic, to Deborah Namm for her vision, and to Scott Laughead, Louise Pielmeier, Tracy Strong, and Mark Lacko for their unflagging encouragement and affection.

Thank you, Steve and Cecile Lindstedt, for laughter, love, philosophy, support, and every succulent fruit of friendship.

And I give my heart, swollen with gratitude, to John Pielmeier, my dear husband, in thanks for his exquisite tenderness and patience, his sterling artistic judgment, and the great sustenance of his love, which is my spirit's daily bread.